Copyright

Copyright © 2023 Andrew Roane

All rights reserved.

No portion of this book may be reproduced in any form without written permission from the publisher or author, except as permitted by U.S. copyright law.

Disclaimer:

Before embarking on any fitness or health program, it is imperative to consult with a qualified healthcare professional or a licensed medical practitioner. The information provided in this book is for general informational purposes only and is not intended as a substitute for professional medical advice, diagnosis, or treatment. The author and publisher of this book are not healthcare professionals, and the content presented here is based on personal experiences, research, and general knowledge available up to the knowledge cutoff date of December 2023. Individual health and fitness needs vary, and what may be suitable for one person may not be appropriate for another.

Readers are encouraged to take responsibility for their health and well-being and to seek the guidance of a qualified healthcare professional before starting any exercise program, making dietary changes, or adopting new health practices. It is crucial to undergo a thorough medical examination to assess one's fitness level and to address any existing health conditions before engaging in physical activities.

The author and publisher disclaim any liability or responsibility for any loss or damage incurred as a direct or indirect result of the use or application of any content presented in this book. Readers should use their discretion and judgment when implementing any health or fitness recommendations and are advised to consult with a healthcare professional to ensure their individual needs and circumstances are taken into account.

Remember that health and fitness are ongoing journeys, and what works for one person may not work for another. Always prioritize your safety and well-being, and make informed decisions based on professional guidance.

Table of Contents

Introduction

5 Fingers of Health and Happiness

The concept of the "5 Fingers of Health and Happiness" integrates principles of personal well-being with a patriotic spirit, emphasizing the interconnectedness of individual health and national prosperity. This approach revolves around the idea that fostering a sense of love for oneself, one's family, and neighbors is crucial for both personal fulfillment and contributing to the greater good of the community. Let's break down the key components of this philosophy:

1. Patriotic Perspective:

- The concept emphasizes the connection between personal health and the well-being of the nation. By maintaining good health, individuals can actively contribute to the overall strength and resilience of their communities and country.

2. Love for Oneself:

- Self-love is foundational to the 5 Fingers of Health and Happiness. It encourages individuals to prioritize their physical, mental, and emotional well-being. This involves practicing self-care, setting boundaries, and cultivating a positive self-image.

3. Love for Family:

- Recognizing the importance of family, this principle encourages individuals to prioritize the health and happiness of their loved ones. Strong familial bonds contribute to a supportive environment that positively influences individual well-being.

4. Love for Neighbors:

- Extending the circle of care beyond the immediate family, the philosophy encourages a sense of community and interconnectedness. Building positive relationships with neighbors and contributing to the well-being of the broader community fosters a harmonious and supportive social environment.

5. Proactive Health and Well-Being:

- The philosophy advocates for a proactive rather than reactive approach to health. This involves adopting a preventive mindset by engaging in regular exercise, maintaining a balanced diet, managing stress, and seeking regular medical check-ups. By taking charge of one's health, individuals can contribute to a healthier, more resilient society.

In summary, the "5 Fingers of Health and Happiness" promotes a holistic approach to well-being that aligns personal health goals with a sense of patriotism and community responsibility. By fostering love for oneself, family, and neighbors, and by adopting a proactive stance towards health, individuals can play an active role in building a healthier, happier, and more resilient society.

Chapter 1 - Nutrition

Nourishing Your Body - The Foundation of Health

In the journey towards health and happiness, Chapter 1 focuses on the cornerstone of well-being: nutrition. This chapter delves into the fundamental elements of a balanced and wholesome diet, emphasizing the importance of fueling your body with the right nutrients for optimal function. Let's explore the key principles of this chapter:

1.1 Protein - Building Blocks for Strength:

- Protein plays a crucial role in the repair and growth of tissues, muscles, and organs. Incorporating lean sources of protein such as poultry, fish, beans, and legumes provides the necessary building blocks for a strong and resilient body.

1.2 Veggies - Nutrient-Rich Powerhouses:

- Vegetables are rich in vitamins, minerals, and antioxidants that support overall health. Embracing a colorful array of vegetables ensures a diverse range of nutrients, contributing to improved immune function, digestion, and vitality.

1.3 Fruit - Nature's Sweet Treats:

- Fruits offer a natural source of sweetness along with essential vitamins and fiber. Including a variety of fruits in your diet not only satisfies your sweet cravings but also provides valuable nutrients that promote heart health and boost energy levels.

1.4 Minimizing Processed Foods - Choose Whole, Real Foods:

- Processed foods often contain added sugars, unhealthy fats, and artificial additives that can negatively impact health. By opting for whole, unprocessed foods, you provide your body with the pure and essential nutrients it needs, reducing the risk of various health issues.

1.5 Cheating Responsibly - Redemption in Choices:

- Acknowledging that occasional indulgences are part of a balanced lifestyle, this chapter encourages a healthy approach to "cheating." If you veer off course, the key is to learn from the experience and make better choices the next day. It's about balance and sustainability rather than strict perfection.

1.6 Say No to Fast Food - Prioritize Your Well-Being:

- Fast food is often laden with unhealthy fats, excessive salt, and empty calories. Avoiding fast food supports both short-term and long-term health goals. Choosing nourishing alternatives reinforces the commitment to your well-being.

1.7 Consistency Over Perfection - Sustainable Habits:

- Recognizing that perfection is an elusive goal, the emphasis is on consistency. Establishing healthy eating habits over time is more sustainable and achievable than striving for flawless adherence. Small, positive choices made consistently lead to significant improvements in overall health.

1.8 Eating Clean - A Commitment to Health:

- "Eating clean" embodies the principle of choosing minimally processed, whole foods. This commitment to clean eating fosters a positive relationship with food, supporting not only physical health but also mental and emotional well-being.

As you embark on your journey toward health and happiness, Chapter 1 lays the foundation by highlighting the significance of nutrition. By focusing on protein, vegetables, and fruits, minimizing processed foods, practicing responsible indulgence, avoiding fast food, and embracing consistency, you pave the way for a nourished and vibrant life.

Chapter 2 - Movement

Energizing Your Body - The Power of Movement and Fitness

In Chapter 2, the spotlight shifts to the vital role of movement and fitness in cultivating health and happiness. This chapter underscores the transformative impact of regular physical activity, promoting a balanced approach that prioritizes daily movement and consistency over an elusive pursuit of perfection. Let's explore the key principles of this chapter:

2.1 Walk, Run, Lift Weights - Embrace Variety:

- Incorporating a diverse range of physical activities ensures a holistic approach to fitness. Whether it's a brisk walk, a rejuvenating run, or the strength-building benefits of weightlifting, variety keeps the body engaged and promotes overall well-rounded fitness.

2.2 Cardio Daily - Boosting Heart Health:

- Cardiovascular exercise, such as running, cycling, or swimming, enhances heart health, improves circulation, and boosts overall stamina. Making daily cardio a part of your routine contributes not only to physical fitness but also to mental clarity and emotional well-being.

2.3 Lift Weights Daily - Building Strength and Resilience:

- Weightlifting is a cornerstone of building muscle strength and endurance. By incorporating daily weightlifting sessions, you not only enhance your physical capabilities but also support bone health, metabolism, and overall functional fitness.

2.4 Consistency Over Perfection - Sustainable Habits:

- Similar to the nutrition chapter, the principle of consistency over perfection applies to fitness. Establishing a daily movement routine, even if it's a short and manageable session, is more sustainable and beneficial in the long run than sporadic, intense workouts.

2.5 Move Every Day - Holistic Wellness:

- Movement goes beyond structured exercise; it encompasses daily activities like walking, stretching, and staying active throughout the day. Prioritizing movement in all aspects of life fosters a lifestyle that supports holistic wellness.

2.6 Daily Movement - Forming Healthy Habits:

- Emphasizing the importance of daily movement, this chapter encourages the formation of healthy habits. Whether it's taking the stairs, going for a short walk during breaks, or practicing quick stretching exercises, consistent movement becomes an integral part of your daily routine.

2.7 Listen to Your Body - Rest and Recovery:

- Attuning to your body's signals is crucial. Rest and recovery are as essential as active movement. Balancing exercise with adequate rest ensures that your body can recover, repair, and adapt, minimizing the risk of overtraining and injuries.

2.8 Mental Benefits - Clarity and Focus:

- Regular physical activity is not only beneficial for the body but also for the mind. It can alleviate stress, enhance mood, and improve cognitive function. Recognizing the mental benefits reinforces the holistic impact of movement on overall well-being.

As you embark on the journey of health and happiness, Chapter 2 highlights the transformative power of movement and fitness. Whether it's walking, running, lifting weights, or embracing daily cardio, the emphasis is on consistency, variety, and listening to your body. By incorporating these principles, you cultivate a lifestyle that energizes both your physical and mental well-being.

Chapter 3 - Sleep

Rejuvenating Your Mind - The Importance of Quality Sleep

In Chapter 3, the focus turns to the often underestimated yet crucial element of well-being: sleep. This chapter underscores the transformative impact of adequate and restful sleep on overall health and happiness. It encourages adopting habits that promote a consistent and quality sleep routine. Let's delve into the key principles of this chapter:

3.1 7 to 9 Hours of Sleep - Prioritizing Rest:

- Recognizing the significance of sleep duration, this chapter emphasizes the goal of getting 7 to 9 hours of sleep each night. Prioritizing sufficient sleep is foundational to physical and mental health, supporting optimal daily functioning.

3.2 Shut Off Devices Early - Creating a Calm Environment:

- Electronic devices emit blue light, which can interfere with the body's natural sleep-wake cycle. The recommendation is to shut off devices at least an hour before bedtime, allowing your mind to transition into a state of relaxation and preparing for restful sleep.

3.3 Dark and Cool Bedroom - Enhancing Sleep Quality:

- Creating an ideal sleep environment involves keeping the bedroom dark and cool. This supports the body's natural circadian rhythm and promotes a comfortable atmosphere conducive to restful sleep.

3.4 Prayer and Meditation - Calming the Mind:

- Engaging in prayer and meditation serves as a powerful tool to calm the mind before sleep. These practices can help alleviate stress, promote mindfulness, and create a sense of inner peace, contributing to a more relaxed transition into sleep.

3.5 Consistency Over Perfection - Establishing a Routine:

- Consistency is once again emphasized as a guiding principle. Establishing a regular sleep routine, including consistent bedtime and wake-up times, helps regulate the body's internal clock, optimizing the quality of sleep over time.

3.6 Wind Down Before Bed - Rituals for Relaxation:

- Incorporating relaxing activities before bedtime, such as reading a book, taking a warm bath, or practicing gentle stretches, signals to your body that it's time to wind down. These pre-sleep rituals contribute to a more gradual and peaceful transition into sleep.

3.7 Mindfulness in Sleep - Quality Over Quantity:

- The chapter underscores the importance of the quality of sleep over sheer quantity. Prioritizing restful, uninterrupted sleep fosters better physical and mental rejuvenation, enhancing overall well-being.

3.8 Napping with Intent - Short and Purposeful:

- While daytime naps can be beneficial, the recommendation is for short and purposeful naps. Keeping them brief and strategic prevents interference with nighttime sleep patterns.

As you navigate the path to health and happiness, Chapter 3 highlights the integral role of sleep. By aiming for 7 to 9 hours of restful sleep, adopting practices to create a conducive sleep environment, and incorporating calming rituals, you enhance the quality of your sleep. The principles of consistency and mindfulness contribute to a holistic approach to well-being that embraces the transformative power of a good night's sleep.

Chapter 4 - Mental Well-Being

Nurturing Your Mind - Cultivating Mental Well-Being

Chapter 4 shifts the focus to the essential aspect of mental well-being, acknowledging the profound impact it has on overall health and happiness. This chapter explores practices and habits that contribute to a positive and resilient mental state, emphasizing the importance of daily self-care. Let's explore the key principles of this chapter:

4.1 Time for Yourself Daily - Self-Care Rituals:

- Prioritizing time for yourself is crucial for mental well-being. Establishing daily self-care rituals, whether it's reading, taking a leisurely walk, or enjoying a hobby, provides a sanctuary for relaxation and personal fulfillment.

4.2 Meditate and Pray - Inner Reflection and Connection:

- Meditation and prayer serve as powerful tools for inner reflection and spiritual connection. These practices not only promote a sense of calm but also provide an opportunity to express gratitude and connect with a higher purpose.

4.3 Gratitude - Appreciating the Present:

- Cultivating gratitude involves acknowledging and appreciating the positive aspects of your life. Regularly expressing gratitude for what you have fosters a positive mindset and shifts focus away from what may be lacking.

4.4 Manifestation - Telling the Universe Your Desires:

- The concept of manifestation involves expressing your desires to the universe. By clearly stating your goals and aspirations, you set a positive intention, aligning your thoughts with your aspirations and inviting positive energy into your life.

4.5 Social Time - Connection with Loved Ones:

- Spending quality time with friends and family is a cornerstone of mental well-being. Social interactions provide support, laughter, and a sense of belonging, contributing to emotional resilience.

4.6 Volunteering - Giving Back to Others:

- Engaging in volunteer activities provides a sense of purpose and fulfillment. Giving back to others fosters a connection with the community and a deeper appreciation for the impact one can have on the lives of others.

4.7 Talking with Friends - Emotional Expression:

- Open communication with friends is vital for mental well-being. Sharing thoughts, concerns, and joys with trusted individuals provides emotional support and strengthens social bonds.

4.8 Consistency Over Perfection - Sustainable Mindful Habits:

- Consistency once again emerges as a guiding principle. Establishing daily habits that nurture mental well-being, such as self-care, gratitude practices, and social interactions, is more sustainable and impactful in the long run than occasional, intense efforts.

4.9 Sunlight: The Vitamins you are missing

- There is growing evidence suggesting a link between vitamin D deficiency and mental health issues. Some studies have shown an association between low vitamin D levels and an increased risk of depression. Vitamin D receptors are present in the brain, and vitamin D is involved in the synthesis of neurotransmitters like serotonin, which plays a role in regulating mood.

As you embark on the journey of health and happiness, Chapter 4 highlights the significance of mental well-being. By incorporating daily practices that prioritize self-care, connection with others, and expressing gratitude, you cultivate a resilient and positive mindset. The principles of consistency and mindfulness contribute to a holistic approach that nurtures not just the body, but also the mind and soul.

Chapter 5 - Proactive Health/Tough Questions

Empowering Your Health - Proactive Engagement with Healthcare

In Chapter 5, the spotlight turns to the pivotal role of proactive engagement in healthcare, emphasizing the responsibility individuals hold for their well-being. This chapter encourages asking tough questions, seeking answers, and actively participating in decisions regarding one's health. Let's delve into the key principles of this chapter:

5.1 Take Responsibility - You Are in Control:

- Acknowledging that a significant portion of health and well-being is within individual control is the first step. By recognizing the role of personal choices, individuals become empowered to take an active role in their health journey.

5.2 Tough Questions for Your Doctor - Open Dialogue:

- Encouraging individuals to engage in open and honest conversations with their healthcare providers, this chapter advocates for asking tough questions. Examples include inquiries about the duration of prescribed medications, potential lifestyle changes, and strategies to reduce or eliminate the need for medication.

5.3 Duration of Medications - Understanding the Plan:

- Asking about the expected duration of prescribed medications opens a dialogue about treatment plans and allows individuals to understand the trajectory of their health journey. This knowledge can guide future decisions about lifestyle changes and proactive health measures.

5.4 Lifestyle Changes - Integrating Health Into Daily Life:

- Inquiring about lifestyle changes necessary for optimal health not only supports the effectiveness of medical interventions but also encourages a holistic approach to well-being. This could involve adjustments in nutrition, fitness, stress management, and other lifestyle factors.

5.5 Nutrition and Fitness - Partners in Health:

- Recognizing the synergy between nutrition, fitness, and overall health, this chapter prompts individuals to explore how lifestyle modifications can positively impact their well-being. This may include personalized plans for diet and exercise to complement medical interventions.

5.6 Seeking Additional Guidance - Building a Support Network:

- If the doctor doesn't have all the answers, asking for recommendations on who to consult reinforces the proactive approach. Building a collaborative network of healthcare professionals ensures a comprehensive and well-informed approach to health.

5.7 Proactive, Not Reactive - A Shift in Mindset:

- Embracing a proactive mindset involves anticipating and addressing health concerns before they escalate. This chapter encourages individuals to view their health journey as a continuous process of improvement and maintenance rather than reacting to issues as they arise.

5.8 Medicine 3.0 - Integrating Personalized Medicine:

- The concept of Medicine 3.0 represents a shift toward personalized and proactive healthcare. This involves tailoring medical interventions to individual needs and incorporating a comprehensive approach that includes lifestyle factors.

As individuals navigate the evolving landscape of healthcare, Chapter 5 highlights the importance of proactive engagement. By asking tough questions, actively seeking information, and integrating lifestyle changes, individuals can play a more significant role in their health and well-being. The principles of responsibility, open communication, and a proactive mindset contribute to a healthcare model that goes beyond treating symptoms to fostering comprehensive, personalized, and sustainable health.

Conclusion

You are in charge of your Health Span Journey!

In conclusion, the journey toward health and happiness is a dynamic and ongoing process. The 5 fingers provide a compass for daily decisions, urging individuals to stay consistent and committed. By being the example, setting positive standards, and embracing proactive health measures, individuals contribute not only to their well-being but also to the well-being of those around them and society at large. The pursuit of health and happiness is not a destination but a continuous, purposeful journey—one that holds the power to transform lives and communities.

Absolutely, it's crucial to emphasize the importance of consulting with healthcare professionals, particularly doctors, before making significant changes to one's exercise routine or prescription medications. Here are some key notes to keep in mind:

1. Consult Your Doctor:

- Always consult with your healthcare provider before making any substantial changes to your exercise regimen or adjusting prescription medications. They can provide personalized advice based on your specific health conditions and needs.

2. Individualized Guidance:

- Your doctor understands your medical history and can offer individualized guidance tailored to your unique circumstances. What works for one person may not be suitable for another, so it's essential to have personalized recommendations.

3. Exercise Modifications:

- Before starting a new exercise program or making significant changes to your current routine, discuss your plans with your doctor. They can assess your fitness level and provide insights into exercises that align with your health goals and any potential limitations.

4. Medication Adjustments:

- If you're considering changes to your prescription medications, whether to reduce or discontinue them, consult your doctor first. Abrupt changes can have unintended consequences, and your healthcare provider can guide you on the safest and most effective way to make adjustments.

5. Holistic Approach:

- This guide serves as a general framework for making healthy daily choices, but it's not a substitute for personalized medical advice. Your doctor can help you integrate these principles into your overall healthcare plan, considering your specific health conditions and needs.

6. Regular Check-Ups:

- Schedule regular check-ups with your doctor to monitor your overall health. These visits provide an opportunity to discuss any changes you're considering and ensure that your health plan aligns with your current well-being.

7. Open Communication:

- Maintain open and transparent communication with your healthcare team. Share your goals, concerns, and any challenges you may be facing. This collaborative approach ensures that your health decisions align with professional medical advice.

8. Safety First:

- Prioritize safety in all health-related decisions. If you experience any adverse effects or unexpected changes in your health, contact your doctor promptly. Your well-being is the top priority, and prompt communication with your healthcare provider is crucial. Remember, your doctor is a valuable partner on your health journey. Their expertise is instrumental in guiding you toward decisions that promote your well-being. Always seek their counsel before making significant changes to your exercise routine or medications. This guide complements, but does not replace, the importance of professional medical advice and supervision.

Bonus Section

Daily Health Enhancers - Optimize health and well-being with these daily

1. Touch the earth. Walk on the earth daily with your shoes off – 3 to 5 minutes.
2. Plunge or cold shower. Get in cool/cold water daily – 3 to 5 minutes.
3. Go for a walk – 15 to 20 minutes.
4. Give a hug and get a hug – 2 minutes.
5. Pray/Mediate/Manifest/Be grateful – 5 to 10 minutes.
6. Stand and face the sun each morning. Get outside. Get real vitamin D. 3 to 5 minutes.
7. Drink plenty of water and hydrogen water if available.
8. Sauna – 20 minutes – 4 to 5 times a week.
9. Eat clean and before 7 pm at night – prioritize protein, veggies and fruit. Natural food. Avoid processed foods.
10. Go to bed – 7 to 9 hours daily.
11. Source your food as local as possible. Meet farmers. Buy Local and eat locally grown food.
12. Floss Daily
13. Limit all screen time
14. Call your family and friends

15. Volunteer and give back.

16. Have a purpose.

Do your on research on all subjects and always consult your health care professionals before making any changes.

Micro Changes – Day 1

1. ______________________________

2. ______________________________

3. ______________________________

4. ______________________________

5. ______________________________

Micro Changes – Day 5

1. ____

2. ____

3. ____

4. ____

5. ____

Micro Changes – Day 10

1. _______________________________

2. _______________________________

3. _______________________________

4. _______________________________

5. _______________________________

Micro Changes – Day 20

1. ____

2. ____

3. ____

4. ____

5. ____

Micro Changes – Day 30

1. ____

2. ____

3. ____

4. ____

5. ____

Micro Changes – Day 60

1. ____

2. ____

3. ____

4. ____

5. ____